I0449819

Situational Survival Guide:

20 Survival Skills To Face Danger And Protect Yourself And Your Family

All photos used in this book, including the cover photo were made available under a Attribution-NonCommercial-ShareAlike 2.0 Generic and sourced from Flickr

Copyright 2016 by the publisher - All rights reserved.

This document is geared towards providing exact and reliable information in regards to the topic and issue covered. The publication is sold with the idea that the publisher is not required to render accounting, officially permitted, or otherwise, qualified services. If advice is necessary, legal or professional, a practiced individual in the profession should be ordered.

- From a Declaration of Principles which was accepted and approved equally by a Committee of the American Bar Association and a Committee of Publishers and Associations.

In no way is it legal to reproduce, duplicate, or transmit any part of this document in either electronic means or in printed format. Recording of this publication is strictly prohibited and any storage of this document is not allowed unless with written permission from the publisher. All rights reserved.

The information provided herein is stated to be truthful and consistent, in that any liability, in terms of inattention or otherwise, by any usage or abuse of any policies, processes, or directions contained within is the solitary and utter responsibility of the recipient reader. Under no circumstances will any legal responsibility or blame be held against the publisher for any reparation, damages, or monetary loss due to the information herein, either directly or indirectly.

Respective authors own all copyrights not held by the publisher.

The information herein is offered for informational purposes solely, and is universal as so. The presentation of the information is without contract or any type of guarantee assurance.

The trademarks that are used are without any consent, and the publication of the trademark is without permission or backing by the trademark owner. All trademarks and brands within this book are for clarifying purposes only and are the owned by the owners themselves, not affiliated with this document.

Table of content

Introduction

Violence seems to be everywhere. If you open a newspaper or switch on the television you will hear about someone who has been attacked. It may be for drugs, money or simply because you have looked at someone the wrong way. It is an unpleasant fact of life that violence could happen at any time. Perhaps even more horrifying is the increase in attacks on those who are most vulnerable. Elderly people and normal families are increasingly falling victim to violent crimes as they are seen as vulnerable.

A violent attack can simply leave you feeling powerless to defend your family and possessions whilst someone helps themselves to what they want. It can emotionally scar you and your family for life; affecting what you feel comfortable doing and even how you approach any situation. These types of situations can even lead to severe physical harm and long lasting, or even life changing injuries. The mental and physical effects of a violent attack can destroy lives long after the physical attack; you may develop post traumatic stress, flashbacks, an inability to leave the house and problems eating and sleeping. In fact, many people simply retreat into a world of their own; no longer able to trust the world around them. One attack can completely change your life and the life of your family.

Fortunately there is a solution. There are several moves which are easy to learn and will help you to defend yourself against an attacker or attackers. Not only will these moves help you to defend yourself, they will also ensure that you can live your life confidently; knowing that you will be able to look after yourself and your family. Violence may be everywhere but there are many things you can do to protect yourself before you even need to use the techniques this book will teach you. It might seem like a situation that you will never find yourself in. However, it can happen to anyone and a little preparation now can make a huge difference to the outcome of any type of aggressive behavior.

In fact, the rules of a violent encounter are simple; wherever possible avoid the situation. This means being aware of what is going on around you, if there is someone who is clearly looking for a fight then there is no shame in giving them plenty of space. Avoiding a situation in the first rule of self defense; why fight if you do not need to?

The second part of any encounter is a follow on; if you have failed to foresee a situation or avoid it then you need to defuse it, if possible. This may not always be possible as it will depend upon your ability to rationalize with the attacker.

Finally, if you are unable to reason with your attacker you will need to be able to defend yourself and your family for long enough to either persuade them to leave or to provide you and your family the opportunity to escape. If you can all get safely away then there is no reason to stay and fight. This stubborn approach can result in your suffering injuries you did not need to receive or, you could even seriously injure your attacker. Whilst this may feel like a desirable ending, it could leave you in trouble with the authorities. In many countries you have the right to defend your property; in fact, in some countries you are even able to kill an attacker on your property if you felt your life was at risk. However, if you do inadvertently injure your attacker, or worse; kill them; you could face an extremely difficult time dealing with the fall out afterwards; this will be far more detrimental to you and your family than the initial attack. Alongside this you may find that you have either over-reacted or are dealing with someone away from your own home; injuring someone who attacks you in this type of situation can result in criminal charges for you!

It is for this reason it is essential to learn the right approach to any potentially violent situation, how to defend yourself and the importance of escaping as soon as you and your family have the opportunity to.

Chapter 1 – Basic Survival techniques

The following techniques are designed to avoid the fight in the first place. These are an important step in self-defense; being able and even willing to fight does not mean you should respond with violence instantly. You have alternative options which can be utilized:

1. **Confidence**

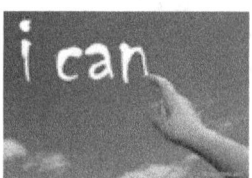

http://www.amazingcoaching.com.au/wp-content/uploads/2015/07/ican.jpg

The majority of people who prey on others can sense who is likely to make an easier victim than others. The aim of most criminals is simply to get in and out with the minimal of fuss. To do this they will choose individuals who are the least likely to fight back. The way to avoid being that victim is to portray an image of confidence and strength; a potential attacker will move onto an easier victim.

You can portray this confidence by walking with your head up, looking others in the eye, without staring and generally being aware of what is going on around you. If you walk with your head up an attacker will find it more difficult to sneak up on you and your body image will project strength. It doesn't matter how you feel inside, your body movements can be enough to dissuade many attackers from seeing you as a victim.

2. **Awareness**

Keeping your head up will also allow you to be more aware of the world around you. The most obvious tip is to avoid areas where there is an increased risk of attack. Why walk through the dark alley unless you really need to! There is more to this than simply avoiding potential trouble spots; sometimes your route will take you through these spots and you must not be afraid to go this way if necessary. You should be sure to improve your awareness of people around you.

The first stage of this is to learn some basic information regarding body postures and how a potential attacker is likely to be stood. They are not likely to be moving with the crowd; instead they will be watching, looking for the easiest victims and making their move quickly and precisely. It is important to note that an attacker does not need to look like a thug; they can be a smartly dressed person.

You need to keep you attention and focus on those around you, how they are moving and if anyone is heading directly for you. This will also ensure you know the ways out of a room or street area as you will be able to see and assess the various escape routes. Remember, you aim is to defend yourself and get out; not put yourself at more risk.

3. **Control**

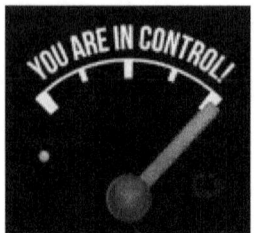

http://milfordandrewpastor.files.wordpress.com/2014/03/control-1.jpg

If an attack and your need to use self defense becomes inevitable then you must learn to control your reactions and the situation you find yourself in. This means being prepared for any issue by knowing the self defense moves in this book. It also means you need to face up to them and adopt a pose from which you are ready to either attack or defend. This will mean standing sideways to minimize your size as a target. One foot needs to be just in front of you, whilst the other should be in-line with your body. This will allow you to move your weight easily and attack or defend according to the attacker's next move.

4. Make a Noise

Before the situation escalates to violence it is essential to raise your voice and challenge your attacker. It is important to keep your voice at an even tone so as not to project fear but also to get as loud as possible. You want other people to know what is happening; you may receive some help or the fact that others are aware of the situation may be enough to persuade your attacker to move on before they attract too much attention. The easiest thing to say to warn the attacker and alert others is simply "Back Off" loudly as you can. Repeating the phrase several times will generate more attention from others.

5. Strike First

If your attempts to warn off your attacker go unheeded and you genuinely believe that you are in imminent danger then you must attack them first. This is when the moves demonstrated later in this book will be of vital importance. Your attack must be aimed at critical areas to ensure you incapacitate your would be attacker as quickly and efficiently as possible. This will reduce the possibility of you becoming injured and will persuade anyone else that it is not worth getting involved.

6. **Where to Hit**

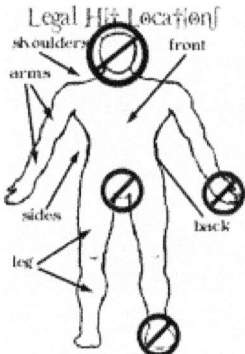

http://mauidotcom.com/images/body2.gif

Once you have decided you must attack, or if you are reacting to their attack then you must move quickly and target areas which will hurt them. At this stage your only concern is inflicting injury which will prevent them from being able or wanting to give chase. This is not a time to adopt a boxing stance or wait to be hit first.

There are several places on the human body which are exceptionally vulnerable; these are the knees, legs, groin and head. In particular the eyes, ears, nose and throat. You will need to hit whichever of these is easiest for you to reach and hit with as much force as possible. This should immediately cause enough injury to allow you to escape. Of course, if you are protecting your family you may need to follow this up with a second or third blow to these vulnerable areas.

7. Rules

It is essential to remember that there are no rules when defending yourself. Your attacker will not adopt a karate or judo stance and expect you to fight them according to the same fighting regime. Indeed, anything can be a weapon and anything you can get your hands on should be used to help protect yourself from an attacker. When your life is at stake then nothing is off limits.

Chapter 2 – 7 Basic Defence techniques

Knowing the places to strike is only the first stage of the fight. To be really effective and decide a fight quickly you need to know the best way to strike any part of an attacker's body. In general you need to use your hand when hitting the upper half of the torso. If you are aiming for the softer parts of the body then a palm strike or holding your hand like a knife will be effective. For tougher parts of the body a tightly curved fist is most effective.

1. **The Eyes**

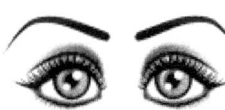

http://pngimg.com/upload/eye_PNG6192.png

The eyes are an extremely vulnerable part of the body; they can be pushed back into their sockets causing pain and extreme discomfort without any permanent damage. If you are close to your attacker then you can gouge, poke or even attempt to scratch your attacker's eyes. Fingers or even your knuckles are the most effective. This is an excellent response when you are facing an attacker who has grabbed one of your arms. The free arm can attack the eyes and your attacker will be stunned by the attack, in pain and potential temporarily blinded or experience blurred vision. This will allow you to escape or, if absolutely necessary, restrain them.

2. The Nose

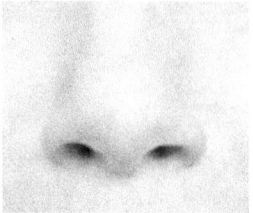

http://www.enhancemyself.com/wp-content/uploads/2015/06/Facts_Nose.jpg

An alternative to the eye gouge when in close quarters is to hit your attacker at the base of their nose. The heel of the palm of your hand should connect with the bottom of their nose. The blow should be aimed at an upward angle and lift their head backwards. It is best to put all your weight behind the blow, this will inflict maximum damage. You are probably aware of how much it hurts when you hit your nose, this amount of force will certainly blur their vision as they eyes will automatically water as the pain shoots upwards. This should be enough to loosen their grip on you.

If your attacker is behind you then you can bring your elbow back and up to connect with the same spot.

3. The Neck

It is easiest to hit the side of someone's neck. This is simply because it is a bigger space than the front and you can connect with the jugular or the carotid artery. Hitting these blood vessels hard can stun your attacker. The most effective way of doing this is to use your hand as a knife. Simply put all your fingers straight and keep them tightly held together. Your thumb should be partially tucked underneath your fingers and bent at the knuckle. Simply extend your arm and swing at the side of the neck with as much force as you can.

If you are not able to hit round the side of their neck then it is possible to hit your attacker in the front of their throat. This can disrupt their breathing and will certainly make them release you. You can opt to bend your fingers at the knuckles and then swing in a straight forward motion; allowing your knuckles to connect with the soft neck tissues. Alternatively you may find it easier to drive your elbow upwards and into their throat. Put the weight of your body behind any blow to cause the maximum damage.

The strength of these types of attack will quickly force your attacker to release you and will ensure that no one else wants to get involved.

4. The Knee

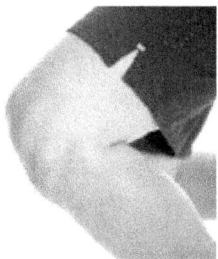

http://www.infinitebodyawareness.com/wp-content/uploads/2015/06/IBA-Hot-Spot-Image-Knee.jpg

Your knee is one of the most vulnerable parts of your body. It is a complicated joint which can easily be disrupted with a sufficient force. Perhaps the best thing about targeting the knee is that it can be hit from any angle and be damaged. In the process it will make it difficult for any attacker to pursue you.

It is worth noting that if you hit the front of the knee you are unlikely to imbalance your attacker; although you are likely to damage their knee more than with any other strike. Losing their balance will automatically ensure they release you. To achieve this you simply need to lift your leg and kick in a downward motion to connect with their knee. Ideally connect with the middle of the base of your foot and hit the side or the back of the knee

5. The Groin

This area of a man's body is particularly sensitive to being hit. However it can also be effective if your attacker happens to be female. The easiest and cleanest strike is to bring your knee up and into the groin. However, for this you need to be directly in front of your attacker facing them. If you are not stood in this position then you may be able to reach their groin with your hand. If you are being attacked by a male then grabbing a handful and squeezing as hard as you physically can, it will have an effect and will certainly force them to release you.

Once released it will be essential to follow up with an additional attack; such as those discussed in the next chapter.

If you are stood a little further back then place all your weight on one leg and swing the other as hard as you can, transferring the weight once you get past the point of no return. Ideally your shin should contact the groin to maximize the initial injury and allow you time to get away.

6. The Headbutt

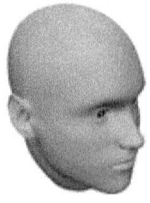

http://www.3dcadbrowser.com/th/1/47/47967.jpg

Funnily the head is one of the most vulnerable areas of your body when being attacked or when defending yourself. However, it is also an exceptionally good weapon! A head butt, properly performed will inflict much more pain on your opponent than it will on you.

The best approach is to grab the collar of an attacker's shirt and push back. They will start to fall and you can jerk them back towards you. This move opens up their shoulders and ensures their arms are out of the way as you bring your head forward.

Following smoothly on from pulling your attacker forward you will need to bring your head forward and down into their face. You should be aiming to connect with their face with the top frontal part of your head. To make sure the right part of you connects your eyes should be focused downwards. This will ensure the right part of your head connects with them and inflicts the maximum amount of pain; potentially breaking their nose and blurring their vision.

7. **The Ear Slap**

This is a very effective technique at off balancing and even temporarily deafening your attacker. It can be used from in front or behind and although most effective with two hands can be completed with just one.

Simply cup your hand and then hit your attacker's ear with all the force you have. Your cupped hand should go flat against their ear, effectively forcing air into their eardrum. If this hit is done hard enough it will rupture their eardrum and leave them disorientated.

If you have both hands free then it can be exceptionally effective to do both ears at the same time; it is highly likely that your attacker will hit the floor as they lose their balance and become dizzy. You can then choose to run or fight; depending upon the situation you find yourself in.

It is worth noting that you are carrying many items which can help in a self defense scenario. Keys can be an exceptionally useful tool; simply slot them between your fingers with the key facing away from you; this will do much more damage than a standard fist. Combs can also be used to push into the upper lift and create a great deal of pain. It is essential to remember than any item which you can put your hand on can be a weapon and it is essential to use it as effectively as possible. When you genuinely believe you are about to be attacked then you must act quickly and decisively.

Chapter 3 – 7 More Advanced Techniques

There are many different self defense moves which can be used by almost anyone. The secret is to learn them and practice them regularly. You do not need to become the ultimate fighter; mastering a few simple moves will allow you to defend yourself if needed. It is much easier to remember the vulnerable areas of the body and have a few basic moves in your repertoire than to attempt to master all the moves you have ever heard of! Knowing a few moves will also allow you to remain calm if attacked. This is an essential part of self defense; remaining calm will allow you to focus on the right move to make and what opportunities are available.

The moves described in the last chapter are attacking moves as a result of being grabbed. This chapter will give you seven techniques which will ensure you are able to initiate the attack before they get a chance:

1. **The Outside Strike**

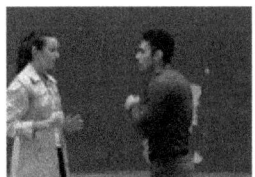

http://greatist.com/sites/default/files/styles/article_main/public/krav_maga_360_defense_0.gif?itok=18b_HBuN

One of the most commonly used punches by many amateur fighters is to swing from with their good arm: usually their right. Their arm will go from a position just behind their buttocks in a swinging motion; aiming to connect with the side of your face. The same movement is used if they intend to slap you or even if they are waving sticks of any sort.

You do not want them to connect with your face and this presents an excellent opportunity to stop them and strike back; hard. Their blow will be stopped by your arm as your fist connects with their chin.

The first thing you need to do is to bring both arms forward slightly bent. Your arm on the same side as the attacker's punch needs to go inside their arm and up. Their blow will then hit your forearm; which is much less damaging than connecting with your face. At the same time that you raise your arm the other hand should be curled into a fist and launch forward at your attacker's face. You need to aim for the previously discussed soft spots; such as the throat or nose. Connecting with the jaw can also be damaging.

It is essential to hit past your target. Do not envision yourself punching their nose; envision yourself punching a spot inside their nose. This will ensure maximum impact.

2. Bear Hugged

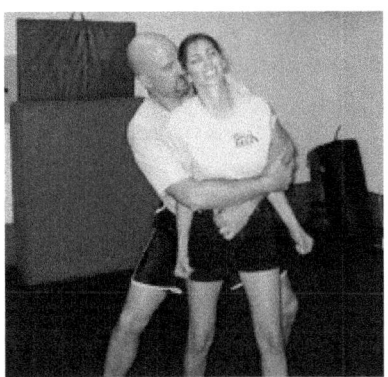

http://www.whatsbestforum.com/attachment.php?attachmentid=9617&d=1367899724

The worst kind of bear hug is when someone grabs you from behind and wraps their arms around your body; keeping your arms trapped inside the hug.

You response should be to instantly push your body downwards, bending your knees as though you are about to do a squat. This dropping motion will lower your sense of gravity and make it difficult for your attacker to continue to hold you or pick you up.

You can follow this by making sure your feet are wider apart then your hips; this will open a pathway to the groin of your attacker. Simply use a knife hand to chop at your attacker's groin. One blow will probably be enough, but if not just keep chopping until they release you.

You can then follow this with a half step forward and then throw all your weight into your elbow; throwing it backwards into your attacker's stomach. As you do this turn around to face them. You can then punch them in the softest parts of the body or simply take the opportunity to escape.

3. The Two handed Choke

One of the worst things about the choke is that a natural response to your air supply being cut off is to panic. This uses your limited air quicker and prevents you from responding effectively. The two handed choke hold can quickly affect your ability to function. It is essential to act fast.

As you feel hands going around your neck, step forward. Then raise your arm on the side that your back leg is. Your arm needs to go up straight so that your bicep is by your ear. Now move your back leg behind your other leg; crossing them over. This will twist your body. Continue the turn as fast as you can with maximum effort. Your bodyweight will be pushing against the wrist of your attacker forcing them to release the hold as you turn. You can then follow with a punch to the nose or even by poking them in the eye.

4. The Solar Strike

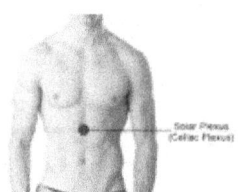

Solar Plexus
(Celiac Plexus)

http://www.buzzle.com/images/health/solar-plexus-location.jpg

Alongside the soft spots on the body there are a few other key areas which can be struck and cause a strong enough reaction to ensure you either escape or have the opportunity to hurt your attacker. The solar plexus is one area that can be hit and will knock the wind out of your attacker's body. This will provide you with the opportunity to follow up with a hit to their nose, throat, eyes or ears.

The solar plexus is located in the centre of the body just below the breast bone. A good punch with curled fist can have even the strongest opponent gasping for air.

Your attacker is likely to bend forward as a reflex in order to catch their breath. This is the perfect opportunity to bring your knee up into their face whilst forcing their head down; this can be achieved by placing both hands behind their head as they move forward. Your momentum will simply be a continuation of their natural reaction.

It is important to practice striking the solar plexus as this will ensure your punch connects with the right spot; you do not want to waste an opportunity to hurt your attacker!

5. **Release your Wrist**

One of the most common ways for an attacker to grab you is to grasp your wrist tight. This can effectively prevent your hand from inflicting any pain on them and even allow them to pull you in the direction they want you to go.

Whilst it is possible to use your free hand to hit them in one of their soft spots, it is also important to know how to release yourself from a wrist hold. This move works regardless of which hand they have grabbed and which of their hands they are using. You can even defeat two wrist holds at the same time.

You will not break their grip by trying to pull away from them. Instead you need to rotate your wrist until your thumb is lined up with the join between your attacker's thumb and his fingers. You can then jerk your arm sharply. This is best achieved by suddenly bending it at the elbow. You will be applying your force to the weakest part of their grip and it will give way; allowing you to escape of fight.

6. **Onslaught**

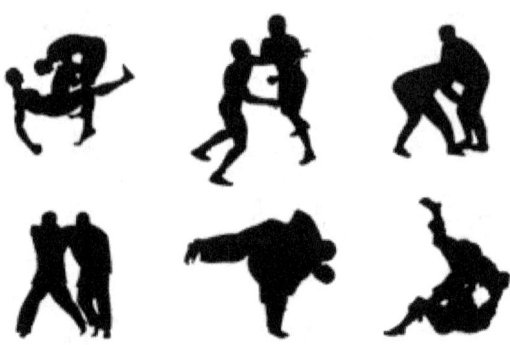

http://www.animation-marseille.ifac.asso.fr/local/cache-vignettes/L376xH221/sitraEVE944781_348237_self-defense-2-eab54.png

One of the worst situations to be caught in is one where there is no obvious escape route and, even if you create one you cannot be sure you will escape as you have others with you that need protecting. In this type of scenario you need to put your attacker down fast to ensure you and your loved one or ones can escape.

To launch an onslaught you need to have your hands up in a defense position and allow your attacker to move towards you. Just before they reach you drop you head and use one arm to block their swing and the other hand should grab their wrist, or forearm. Keep your head tucked behind your blocking arm as you reach behind their neck; moving your body to the side; forcing one of their arms put wide. As you move to the side place your hand on the back of their neck and push downwards; simultaneously lifting the arm that is holding their forehand. Your attacker will be forced downwards and the upwards movement of his other arm will cause him to flip. His free hand will hit the floor to stop him from hurting himself leaving his other arm between your grip and your arm; effectively immobilizing him. From her you can drag him; punch his neck or even drop an elbow into his solar plexus or groin to ensure he doesn't want to get back up.

7. **The Grapple**

It is vital to stay on your feet if at all possible. This means being mindful of any attempt to take your legs away. Your attacker may reach for your legs. The first thing you must do is move back to prevent them from either getting a good grip or any grip. Your attacker will be crouched aiming for your legs meaning that the back of their neck will be exposed. It is possible to drive your elbow into their neck; however, if you miss you are leaving yourself vulnerable. A safer technique is to twist your body so that you are side to side, your forearm will go against his head forcing him away from your legs. You can then twist one hundred and eight degrees to connect a punch with his jaw. It is even possible to follow this up by driving your knee upwards into his face.

Conclusion

Self defense is an important subject that everyone should take the time to learn a little about. It is one skill that you hope you will never need to use but will be exceptionally grateful for it if you do find yourself in that sort of situation. To ensure you will react properly you need to be confident in your abilities. This means practicing so that the basic moves are remembered and even become automatic. To do this it is essential to find a friend who is willing to practice with you and you will both benefit from learning these valuable skills.

Many people will attempt to learn as many different techniques and moves as possible; believing this will help them to deal with any attack that they experience. However, the more moves you have in your repertoire the more difficult it will be for your mind to make a snap decision as to which approach is best or which move to use. Unless you are training to become a professional fighter then it is better to learn a few basic techniques and moves which will enable you to handle any situation. It is also important not to believe that the only way to win is to beat the attacker up. Unfortunately this is likely to see you facing criminal charges! You should use enough force to allow you to escape; this will ensure you remain on the right side of the law. A successful outcome means that you have survived, preferably without any injury.

As already mentioned it is also important not to forget that there are no rules in real fighting. Anything which you can put your hand on can be used as a weapon to fight your opponent. Even if you are fortunate enough to be carrying a gun, you will need to be a reasonable distance from your attacker to have time to get it and remove the safety before you can fire. Experts estimate that anyone closer than twenty one feet will get to you before you can fire the gun. If they are twenty one feet away you probably already have a good escape option available.

The real secret to self defense is to be prepared and vigilant. Spotting potential trouble before it happens allows you to stay clear of any danger areas and avoid the need to fight or defend yourself. Of course, this is not always possible but an awareness of your surroundings will help you know what options are available to you.

Finally, no matter how good your fighting experience or your belief in your own techniques; if there are four or five blokes and they want your wallet which has a small amount of money in it; it is better to give it to them than to fight and be injured. A small amount of money is not worth it and you can easily cancel the cards in your wallet. Keep it simple and you will survive to win another battle; your life is worth much more than any number of possessions.

FREE Bonus Reminder

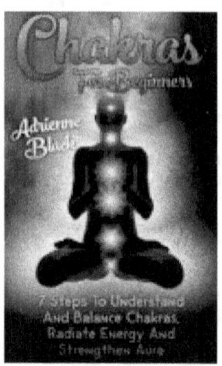

If you have not grabbed it yet, please go ahead and download your special bonus E book *"Chakras for Beginners. 7 Steps To Understand And Balance Chakras, Radiate Energy, And Strengthen Aura"*.

Simply Click the Button Below

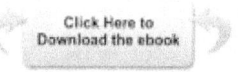

OR Go to This Page

http://lifehacksworld.com/free

BONUS #2: More Free & Discounted Books & Products

Do you want to receive more Free/Discounted Books or Products?

We have a mailing list where we send out our new Books or Products when they go free or with a discount on Amazon. Click on the link below to sign up for Free & Discount Book & Product Promotions.

=> Sign Up for Free & Discount Book & Product Promotions <=

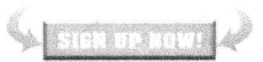

OR Go to this URL

http://zbit.ly/1WBb1Ek

www.ingramcontent.com/pod-product-compliance
Lightning Source LLC
Chambersburg PA
CBHW061950280526
45787CB00004B/1797